Instant Pot Cookbook
Instant Pot Recipes for Weight Loss

Table of Content

Creamy Coleslaw with Pressure Cooker Ribs

Conclusion

Introduction

I want to thank you and congratulate you for downloading the book, *"Instant Pot Cookbook: Instant Pot Recipes for Weight Loss"*. This book contains proven steps and strategies on how to use instant pot in a tactical way and make different types of finger kinking food, which are also paleo friendly. Why you should use instant pot and some unique hack that are very surprising is written here very easily so that you can easily make dishes with your instant pot. I hope you will enjoy the book, as there is all about you want to know.

Thanks again for downloading this book, I hope you enjoy it!

Chapter 1: Instant Pot: Is it worth?

- ➢ It makes meat cook the easiest thing ever, and you do not need to plan more. You can even include some additional cook time and cook froze meat without having to defrost it.

- ➢ It makes prepping and cooking your own bone soup as easy as it gets because you can make it in only a couple of hours instead of 24 or more.

- ➢ You can set your meal to cook and after that abandon it on the "keep warm" setting with the goal that it's prepared and waiting when you return home from work, for up to 10 hours.

- ➢ You can utilize it to make your own particular coconut yogurt significantly more speedily than waiting for yogurt to culture the traditional way.

- ➢ The top of the Instant Pot can be cleaned with foamy water, but ought not to be set in the dishwasher.

- ➢ The sealing ring can be expelled from the top and is easily cleaned after a fast suds and wash — it isn't usually caked with food.

- ➢ You can batch cook enough baby food in a couple of hours to bolster your kid for a month or longer. Bonus: Pressure-cooking retains a greater number of nutrients than boiling or roasting in the oven, which is likely best used when you are making food for your little one.

- I have been asked if the Instant Pot requires any "unique" cleaning, and I need to state, it's easy to keep in your kitchen.

- The inner, removable stainless steel pot tidies up easily with a swift soap and water douse, and is dishwasher safe.

- You can utilize it as a slow cooker, so it enables you to eliminate a massive kitchen machine from your cabinets, although I don't know why you would decide on slow cooking versus instant cooking with its suitable keep warm feature.

- The bigger, external portion of the Instant Pot is the same as any crockpot casing, and should simply be wiped down with a wet cloth.

Chapter 2: Awesome Hacks to Make You Love Your instant pot

1. Better hard-boiled eggs than you've at any point made before. Tired of your hard-boiled eggshells not peeling away? Never know the right approach to cook them? Find out the best hack for cooking hard-boiled eggs in the Instant Pot. You'll never attempt stovetop eggs again.

2. Make your own particular applesauce that is healthier than store-purchased. Oh! One minute. Did I neglect to mention you could do it in 3 minutes?

3. Prompt homemade stock. You have presumably heard about the amazing health advantages of bone broth. If you're cooking meat on the bone, simply include water and turn it into homemade broth over minutes.

4. Freeze your leftovers in round containers.

5. Generally, when you make a freezer feast or soup, you utilize freezer bags and lay them flat. Instead, fill your freezer bags with your leftovers and after that put the bag into a round container. The bag will solidify in a cylinder form which you can then slip into the Instant Pot and have a warm dinner in minutes.

6. Dispose of the stinky ring smell. The one downfall of the Instant Pot that I've experienced is that the silicone-sealing ring assimilates all of the odors

you are cooking. Nobody needs curry mixed with their applesauce. You can purchase new ones, or simply soak it a mixture of vinegar and boiling water or baking soda and high temperature hot water.

7. Goodness my-kettle corn in the Instant Pot. What can this machine not do? I'd never thought of popping popcorn in the Instant Pot, but you can! I bet you could even attempt our most loved kettle corn Instant Pot style too.

8. You can make perfect jam.

9. Crazy but real... you can make doggy food in your Instant Pot. Save money on the store-purchased version of your hairy companion's most loved food and make your own.

10. Who knew? You can even make hard lotion. What is hard lotion? It is a solid bar of lotion (not to be confused with soap) that stays strong at room temperature and can be applied to dry hands, feet, and body. Unlike liquid lotions, it's all natural and yes, siree can be made in the Instant Pot!

11. Plan for a longer cooking time. Mostly, your Instant Pot takes about 5 - 10 additional to warm up and chill off.

12. Sauté away! Try not to pass up a great opportunity for the sauté feature of the Instant Pot... it is incredible! Include somewhat olive or coconut oil to the bottom of the pot, fill it with veggies or meat, and it sautés like any frying dish.

13. Simple homemade yogurt. If you've ever thought of making your own particular yogurt, the Instant Pot is the place to do it.

14. Supplant your oven with the Instant Pot. Practically anything you cook in the oven can be cooked in the Instant Pot (stuffed peppers are wonderful!). Simply cut the cooking time down to 1/3.

15. After you cook meats, utilize the "Sauté" setting to diminish and stew sauces or to make gravy.

16. Supplant your microwave. You can diminish your experience to your microwave's radiation by reheating food in your Instant Pot. Utilize the "Slow Cook" or "Keep Warm" features.

17. Make your own delightful vanilla extract.

18. Yap! Pasta works in the pressure cooker! The noodles cook snappier than you can imagine and you can even make one-pot pastas that's cool.

19. Perfect cheesecake in the Instant Pot.

20. Child pleasing mac and cheddar in 10 minutes. In addition, I'm not talking the powdered kind. This version is velvety, marvelous, and kid-approved.

21. Include ½ cup of water {almost} all time. Your pressure cooker depends on steam and internal heat to cook your foods. Most foods require at least ½ cup of water, broth, or other fluid to adequately cook foods.

22. Now this is amazing… make your own 100% natural cough syrup in the Instant Pot!

Chapter 3: Recipes

Below is a section of our favorite air fryer recipes. Explore these dishes and enjoy!

Instant Pot Roasted Potatoes

Servings 4 persons, Preparation time 5 minutes, cooking time: 15 minutes

Ingredients:

- ¼ cup avocado oil, olive oil, or ghee

- ½ teaspoon onion powder

- ¼ teaspoon paprika

- ¼ teaspoon ground black pepper

- 1 teaspoon garlic powder

- 1 teaspoon (or more) sea salt

- 1.5 pounds russet potatoes

- 1 cup chicken broth

Directions:

1. Slice the potatoes into wedges

2. Plug in your Instant Pot and press "Sauté"

3. Add in the cooking fat and enable it to heat up

4. Cautiously include the potatoes and cook them for 5-8 minutes, shifting them as they cook

5. Sprinkle the seasonings, pour in the stock and press the "Cancel/Off" button

6. Secure the lid, cut off the pressure valve, and press the "Manual" button

7. Press the "- " button until your chance show peruses 7 minutes

8. Let them to cook and after that brisk release the steam once finished

9. Let the steam exit totally and after that evacuate the top

10. Season with a touch of additional ocean salt if required

Pina Colada Chicken - AIP & Paleo

Servings 4 persons, Preparation time 15 minutes, cooking time: 15 minutes

Ingredients:

- 1/8 teaspoon salt

- 2 tablespoons coconut aminos

- ½ cup full fat coconut cream (see note to make your own)

- 1 teaspoon cinnamon

- 2 pounds Organic chicken thighs, cut into 1" chunks

- 1 cup fresh or frozen pineapple chunks

- ½ cup chopped green onion (garnish)

Directions:

1. Place all ingredients, except green onions, into Instant Pot.

2. Close lid.

3. Press Poultry button.

4. Pot will automatically set itself for 15 minutes, high pressure.

5. Let to cook.

6. Once cooking has stopped, do off Instant Pot.

7. Let pressure release naturally for 10 minutes.

8. Carefully open lid and expel from pot.

9. Stir.

10. If you would like to thicken the sauce a bit, essentially stir in a teaspoon of arrowroot starch blended with a tablespoon of water.

11. Then, press the Sauté button.

12. Cook until sauce thickens to your liking.

13. Now Turn off Instant Pot.

14. Serve with green onion decorate.

Beef Stew (Paleo, Grain-Free)

Servings 8 persons, Preparation time 10 minutes, cooking time: 45 minutes

Ingredients:

- onion powder
- pound Grass-fed beef stew meat approximately
- Organic Coconut Oil
- a few yukon gold potatoes diced
- turmeric
- chipotle powder
- salt & pepper
- 1 large onion diced
- 3 stalks celery chopped
- garlic powder
- 2 Tbsp arrowroot powder dissolved in 2 Tbsp cool water
- paprika
- 2 c homemade stock (chicken beef, or veggie)
- 3-5 carrots peeled and chopped
- frozen peas

Directions:

1. Turn the instant pot to "sauté" and include a couple tablespoons of coconut oil.

2. When the pot is warm, add the stew meat and brown on both sides.

3. Include 1 cup of stock, and secure the lid. Ensure the vent is shut.

4. Turn the pot off, at that point on "manual" (high pressure) for 20 minutes.

5. When the pot beeps those 20 minutes is over, do a snappy release of the steam, and open the pot.

6. Add the majority of the vegetables except for the peas, whatever is left of the stock, and sprinkle in flavors to taste. Stir to mix.

7. Supplant the lid and close the steam exhaust. Set the pot on "manual" (high pressure) for another 10 minutes.

8. When the pot beeps, let it sit for another 10 minutes (the pot checks up, to enable you to follow along), then speedy release whatever remains of the steam.

9. Stir in the arrowroot slurry to set the broth a bit, and include however many solidified peas you like. The peas will defrost and be warmed by the hot stew without getting soft or overcooked.

Cauliflower Soup with Creamed Fennel

Servings 4 persons, Preparation time 15 minutes, cooking time: 15 minutes

Ingredients:

For the salad:

- ➤ 1 tablespoon coconut oil
- ➤ 1 cup coconut milk
- ➤ 3 cups broth (bone broth or vegetable broth)
- ➤ 2 teaspoons salt
- ➤ 1 white onion
- ➤ 3 cloves garlic
- ➤ 1 extra-large or 2 medium sized fennel bulbs, stalks and fronds removed
- ➤ 1 pound cauliflower florets
- ➤ Optional: Truffle oil, for serving
- ➤ Optional: Black pepper for serving (note: this recipe is AIP-friendly if you skip the pepper).

Directions:

1. Slice the onions, mince the garlic, and cleave the fennel. If your cauliflower is not as of now slashed into florets, do that now. In the bottom of your pressure cooker, warmth ups the coconut oil. Sauté the onions until luminous. Include the garlic, fennel, and cauliflower. Sauté for 5-10 minutes, until the edges of the vegetables begin to turn golden.

2. Pour the broth and coconut milk into the pot. Include salt. Cook on the soup setting for at least 5 minutes.

3. Once the pressure cooker is done cooking, release the pressure and evacuate the lid. Utilize a standing blender or an immersion blender to puree the soup to a smooth, soft consistency.

4. Scoop into serving dishes and sprinkle with truffle oil. Top with newly saltine pepper, and topping with a left over fennel frond. Serve warm.

Cherry Tomato Chicken Cacciatore

Servings 6 persons, Preparation time 5 minutes, cooking time: 15 minutes

Ingredients:

- 1 pound (500g) cherry tomatoes
- 1 cup water
- 1 sprig fresh basil leaves, torn
- 2 garlic cloves, crushed.
- ¼ teaspoon hot pepper flakes (or one fresh hot pepper, chopped)
- 1 teaspoon salt (use 2 teaspoons if your chicken has not been previously salt-brined)
- 1 teaspoon olive oil
- 3 pounds (1.5 kilos) bone-in chicken legs and thighs
- 1 teaspoon dried oregano ¼ cup (60ml) tart red table wine (such as Merlot)
- ½ cup (70g) pitted green olives, rinsed

Directions:

In the heated pressure cooker, add the olive oil and brown the chicken thighs on all sides. In the meantime, expel the stems from the cherry tomatoes and place them in a big ziploc pack so they are in a single layer. Close the pack totally - leave a tiny opening at the end. Alternatively, on the other lightly tie a common plastic bag. With a meat pounder, or hefty pot, softly squash the all part of the cherry tomatoes - the aim is to burst them open, not crush them. Put the chicken aside and pour the pounded cherry tomato blend and the greater part of its juice into the pressure cooker base. Include the garlic, hot pepper, salt, oregano, wine and water and blend well, scraping up the brown bits of chicken adhered to the bottom of the cooker. Place the chicken over into the pressure cooker and blend to coat the chicken with the contents of the cooker. At that point, "smooth" out the chicken pieces into an even layer. Close and bolt the lid of the pressure cooker. For electric pressure cookers: Cook for 13-14 minutes at high pressure. For stove top pressure cookers: Turn the heat up to high and when the cooker indicates it has achieved high pressure, lower to the heat to continue it and begin counting 12 minutes pressure cooking time. At the point when time is up, open the cooker by freeing the pressure through the valve. Mix the contents and let the cooker stand unlidded for about 5 minutes, stirring infrequently to lessen some of the cooking fluid using the pressure cooker's lingering heat. Using a slotted spoon, lift into a serving casserole and sprinkle with green olives and basil before serving. Keep the broth, left in the base of the pressure cooker to use set up of stock in a risotto or rice recipe.

Chicken Shredded Pressure Cooker

Servings 6 persons, Preparation time 10 minutes, cooking time: 10 minutes

Ingredients:

- ➤ ½ cup water or chicken broth
- ➤ 1 teaspoon salt
- ➤ 4 pounds chicken breast
- ➤ ½ teaspoon black pepper

Directions:

1. Add all the ingredients to the instant pot.

2. Lid with the top, close the pressure valve, and set the ideal opportunity for 20 minutes at high pressure.

3. Once the pressure cooking time has finished, deliberately turn the valve from "sealing" to "venting" to fast pressure discharge. (This will enable the steam to escape and you'll be ready to open the top sooner than waiting for natural release).

4. Place the chicken onto a plate or cutting board and utilize two forks to shred.

5. Store the chicken in an air free container with the fluid to help keep the meat moist.

Instant Pot Carrots Sweet and Spicy

Servings 4, Preparation time: 10 minutes, cooking time: 10 minutes

Ingredients:

- ➢ 1 teaspoon Paprika
- ➢ 1 cup water
- ➢ 2 teaspoons Ground Mustard
- ➢ 1 lb carrots
- ➢ ¼ cup Organic Blackstrap Molasses
- ➢ 2 tablespoons Butter
- ➢ 1 teaspoon Cumin
- ➢ 2 teaspoons minced Garlic
- ➢ 2 tablespoons Stone Ground or Yellow Mustard
- ➢ Hot Sauce (to taste)
- ➢ Salt and Pepper (to taste)

Directions:

1. Cut your carrots the long way into quarters-and cut those down the middle if require be.

2. Add one cup of water to the Instant Pot, at that point include the trivet or steam basket, and at that point include your carrots. Put the lid on; ensure the valve is set to sealing.

3. Set the Instant Pot for Manual – High – 1 Minute. Release the pressure using the fast release technique.

4. Carefully put aside the carrots (which ought to be completely cooked through-you can test with a fork), and dump out the water.

5. Set the Instant Pot to Sauté.

6. Add in butter and molasses. At the point when the butter has softened, include the remaining ingredients-and mix.

7. When everything is very much blended (should not take over a minute or something like that) off the Instant Pot and include the carrots once more into the pot.

8. Stir to coat the carrots with the sauce blend.

Swift Onion Soup AIP

Servings 4, Cooking time: Preheat – 10 minutes, cooking time – 8 minutes

Ingredients:

- ➢ 2 bay leaves

- ➢ 1 tbsp / 15 ml balsamic vinegar

- ➢ 2 tbsp / 30 ml avocado oil, coconut oil or good quality lard

- ➢ 6 cups / 1.4 L pork stock

- ➢ 1 tsp / 5 g real salt

- ➢ 8 cups / 960 g yellow onions

- ➢ 2 large sprigs of fresh thyme

Direction

1. Cut the onions down the middle through the root, peel them, and cut them into thin half-moons. Set the Instant Pot to "Sauté" and include the oil. Once the oil is hot, include the onions. Cook the onions until they have lessened down and become translucent, stirring sometimes to anticipate sticking, about 15 minutes.

2. Add the balsamic vinegar and rub up any fond from the bottom of the Instant Pot, at that point include the stock, salt, straight leaves and thyme. Do off the Instant Pot and close the lid of the Instant Pot, making beyond any doubt to watch that the float is free and the vent is not congested and that the lid is set in the "Sealing" place.

3. Set the Instant Pot to "High Pressure" and cook the soup for 10 minutes once it has come up to pressure. Enable the strain to release using the

"natural release" - don't open the vent or hot fluid may spout out of the vent along with the steam.

4. Discard the bay leaves and thyme stems; at that point mix the soup together using an immersion blender either specifically in the pot, or by moving the soup deliberately to a blender.

Beet Borscht

Servings 4, Preparation time: 10 minutes, cooking time: 10 minutes

Ingredients:

- ½ tbsp thyme
- 3 large beets peeled, or 8 cups diced
- 3 cups shredded cabbage
- 6 cups stock, (beef, chicken or veggie)
- Bay leaf
- 1 tbsp salt
- 1 medium onion diced
- 3 stalks celery diced, or ½ cup
- ¼ cup chopped fresh dill
- 2 large cloves garlic diced
- 2 large carrots diced, or ½ cup
- ½ cup Coconut yogurt or sour cream (optional)

Directions:

1. Place washed beets in a steamer in the instant pot with 1 cup of water. Steam for 7 minutes, fast release, and drop into an ice bath, the skins will slip right off! Chop.
2. Add: beets, carrots, celery, garlic, onions, cabbage, inlet leaf, stock, salt, and thyme to the instant pot.
3. Press the "Soup" setting adjusting the chance to 45 minutes.

4. Let a natural pressure release or else it's soup splashing all over)

5. Spoon into bowls adding a spot of sour cream and garnish with fresh dill

Chili Instant Pot Habanero

Servings: 3 persons, Preparation time: 15 minutes, Cooking Time: 15 minutes

Ingredients:

- ➢ 1 tablespoon chili powder
- ➢ 1 onion, diced
- ➢ 3 stalks celery, chopped
- ➢ 2 (14.5 ounce) cans organic diced tomatoes
- ➢ 2 teaspoons oregano
- ➢ 4-5 cloves garlic, minced
- ➢ 1 habanero, minced (use 2 if you like your food insanely spicy)
- ➢ 1 bell pepper, chopped
- ➢ 5 medium carrots, chopped
- ➢ 1 tablespoon avocado oil
- ➢ 1 pound ground beef
- ➢ 1 ½ teaspoon cumin powder
- ➢ 1 teaspoon salt, adjust to taste
- ➢ 1 teaspoon paprika
- ➢ Beef Bacon, cooked and crumbed (optional)

Directions:

1. Press the "Sauté" button on the Instant Pot, and include the oil, onions, and garlic. Sauté for 2 minutes, at that point add the ground beef to the pot and cook until it become brown.

2. Add the remaining ingredients, blend well, at that point lid, and bolt the lid. Press the "Keep Warm/Cancel" button on the Instant Pot, at that point press the "Meat/Stew" button to begin the pressure-cooking. It will mechanically be set for 35 minutes. Confirm the steam valve is shut.

3. Once the bean stew is done, the Instant Pot will routinely change to the "Keep Warm" mode. Enable the strain to release naturally or utilize the speedy release.

4. Top with disintegrated bacon if wanted and serve.

Grass Fed Back Beef Ribs

Servings: 2 persons, Preparation time: 10 minutes, Cooking Time: 15 minutes

Ingredients:

- ¾ cup water

- 4 ounces of unsweetened apple sauce

- 1 rack of grass fed beef back ribs (~ 3.5 pounds)

- Dry rub of choice (I used Penzeys Chili 9000)

- Kosher salt

- 2 tablespoons coconut aminos

- 1 teaspoon fish sauce

Directions:

1. Snatch a rack of grass fed beef back ribs and pat them dry with a paper towel. At that point, sprinkle it liberally on both sides with the dry rub and kosher salt.

2. Wrap it up in thwart to marinate for at least two hours and up to a day.

3. When you're prepared to cook the ribs, preheat the broiler with the rack positioned 4-6 inches from the heating module.

4. Snatch the rack from the freeze and cut it so it'll fit in your pressure cooker. If you have a 6-quart pot, cut the rack into three even pieces. Put the ribs on a wire rack in a thwart lined, rimmed baking sheet.

5. Sear the ribs for 1-2 minutes on each side to get a pleasant burn. Keep the grill on because you'll be broiling these meaty bones again at the end.

6. Include the water, apple sauce, coconut aminos, and fish sauce to the pressure cooker. Mix to combine and add a rack to the pot.

7. Heap the ribs into the pressure cooker and bolt on the lid.

8. Wrench the heat to high and when the pot achieves high pressure, turn down the heat to maintain high pressure on the most reduced setting conceivable. Cook on high pressure for 20 minutes and let the pressure descend naturally or release it rapidly.

9. Evacuate the ribs and place them back on a wire rack atop a thwart lined, rimmed baking sheet.

10. Stew the cooking fluid until it is lessened to 2 cups (~5 minutes). Skim off the abundance fat at the top if wanted and alter seasoning.

11. Baste the racks with the braising fluid…

12. … In addition, cook them for about a minute to get some crusty bits.

13. With a least investment in time, you will got yummy delicate ribs.

Blueberry Jam in Easy Instant Pot

Servings: 2 persons, Preparation time: 10 minutes, Cooking Time: 110 minutes

Ingredients:

- ➢ 1 pound (500g) honey, preferably local
- ➢ 2 pounds (1kg) blueberries, fresh or frozen

Directions:

1. Add blueberries to inner pot of pressure cooker.
2. Pour in honey.
3. Put pressure cooker on low heat (Keep Warm function if using Instant Pot or other electric cooker) until honey melts. If using solidified berries, this part may take a while, but do not stress.
4. Stir occasionally.
5. When softened, turn pressure cooker to high heat (Sauté function on Instant Pot) until honey simmers. There will be white-pink air pockets all around the strawberries.
6. When it boils, rapidly put on the top of your cooker, checking that the seals and all components are well, including being in the sealing position.
7. If using an electric cooker, hit the Cancel button, at that point set too high for 2 minutes.
8. If using a stovetop cooker, bring to high pressure and maintain pressure for a cook time of 2 minutes.

9. When cooking time is over, if using an electric cooker, hit the Cancel button to off the heat, and unplug.

10. With a stovetop cooker, expel from heat.

11. Let depressurize naturally.

12. When depressurized, evacuate lid and play Judas on to high heat (Sauté function on Instant Pot).

13. Let boil until some of the water has evaporated off, and the stick is pleasant and gelled when trickled off a spoon. Make a point to rub the bottom every now and again to ensure anyhow gelling.

14. Pour jam into clean half-pint containers.

15. Store in the refrigerator.

Creamy Coleslaw with Pressure Cooker Ribs

Servings: 4 persons, Preparation time: 30 minutes, Cooking Time: 35 minutes

Ingredients:

- ½ tsp. garlic powder
- 1 tsp. onion powder
- ¾ tsp. black pepper
- ½ tsp. paprika
- ½ tsp. salt
- 2.5 lbs. baby back ribs
- ½ tsp. dry mustard
- ½ tsp. chili powder

Ingredients for the BBQ sauce

- ¾ cup tomato sauce
- ⅓ cup apple cider vinegar
- ½ tsp. smoked paprika
- ¼ cup + 1 tbsp coconut aminos
- 2 slices bacon, finely chopped
- ½ tsp. cayenne pepper
- 6 oz. tomato paste
- ½ cup all natural apple juice
- ½ onion, finely chopped
- 2 garlic cloves, minced
- Sea salt and freshly ground black pepper

- ➢ 1 tbsp cooking fat

Ingredients for the coleslaw

- ➢ 1 cup red cabbage, shredded (about ¼ of a head)
- ➢ 2 carrots, shredded
- ➢ 2 green onions, finely chopped
- ➢ 3 cups green cabbage, shredded (about ½ of a head)
- ➢ 1 cup raisins
- ➢ 2 ½ tsp caraway seeds
- ➢ ¾ cup homemade mayonnaise
- ➢ ¼ cup apple cider vinegar
- ➢ Sea salt and pepper to taste

Directions:

1. Add the cabbage, carrots, green onions, and raisins to a substantial mixing dish.

2. In a separate littler bowl, combine the caraway seeds, mayonnaise, apple juice vinegar, salt, and pepper.

3. Add the dressing to the cabbage and vegetables and blend to combine.

4. Lid and refrigerate until prepared to serve.

5. Next influence the dry rub for the ribs by mixing the onion to powder, dark pepper, paprika, salt, dry mustard, garlic powder, and bean stew powder.

6. Cut the ribs into chunks or individual pieces so they fit inside the pressure cooker. Stacking them is all right, so in many cases cutting the racks into thirds ought to be sufficient. Coat the ribs done with the dry rub.

7. Add the minimum measure of water required for the pressure cooker (consult the manual), include the cooking rack, and after that place the ribs inside, stacking them freely. Place the top on the pressure cooker and cook at high pressure for 15 minutes. In the interim, make the bbq sauce by heating the cooking fat in a sauté container over a medium heat.

8. Once hot, include the bacon and cook until fresh.

9. Next include the garlic and onion and sauté for 5 minutes, or until the onions soften. Include the remaining ingredients for the bbq sauce and mix well.

10. Bring to a boil, at that point diminish the heat and let stew for 5-10 minutes.

11. Once the ribs have cooked for 15 minutes, deliberately release the pressure and expel the top. Exchange the ribs to a plate. Evacuate the cooking rack and dispose of any fluid from the cooking pot.

12. Add some bbq sauce to the bottom of the pressure cooker, enough to lid, at that point include a layer of ribs, and include more sauce, at that point another layer of ribs et cetera so the ribs are stacked and all lidded in sauce.

13. Return the top to the pressure cooker and cook on high pressure for another 10 minutes.

14. After 10 minutes release the pressure and exchange the ribs to a serving plate.

15. Serve warm with the coleslaw on the side.

Conclusion

Thank you again for downloading this book! I hope this book was able to help you to cook tactically in your instant pot. The shorter cooking times related with pressure-cooking are supposed to reserve nutrients and taste better than consistent scorching. The meals I have made with it so far have been quite delightful and the component makes it comparatively easy to vapor things using the comprised steaming stand and the large, flexible-to-wash container. I hope that you'll also experience the same thing when you'll use it. Best of luck and Happy cooking.

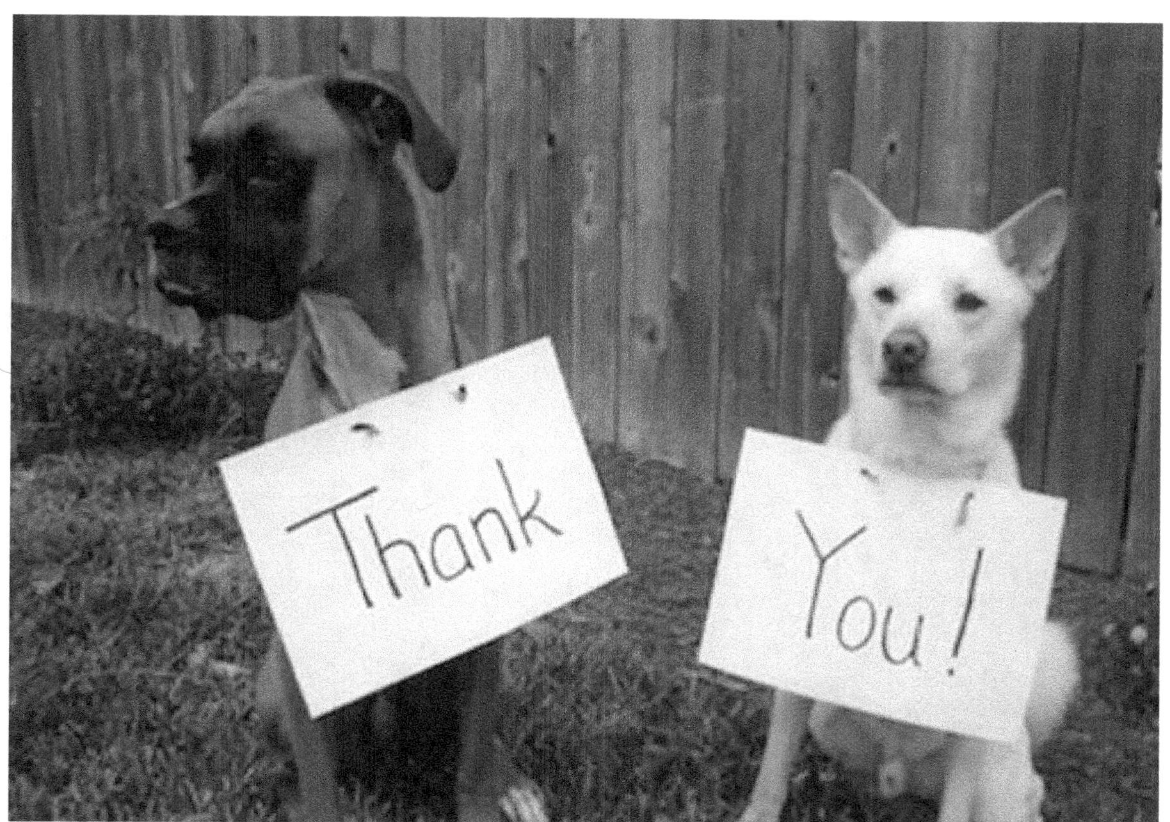

Finally, if you enjoyed this book, then I'd like to ask you for a favor, would you be kind enough to leave a review for this book on Amazon? It would be greatly appreciated!

Click here to leave a review for this book on Amazon!

Thank you and good luck!

Preview Of 'Air Fryer Cookbook'

Chapter I: Fry without Fat! Incredible Ways to Prepare Healthy Food Using Air-Fryer

- Find the perfect place for your air fryer in your kitchen. Continuously keep your air fryer on a level, heat-safe countertop and ensure there are at least five inches of space behind the air fryer where the fumes vent is located.

- Pre-heat your air fryer before adding your food. This is easy – simply turn the air fryer on to the temperature that you need and set the clock for 2 or 3 minutes. At the point when the clock goes off, the air fryer has pre-heated and is prepared for food.

- Invest in a kitchen splash bottle. Spraying oil on the food is easier than drizzling or brushing, and enables you to utilize less oil overall. While you can purchase oil sprays in cans, sometimes there are aerosol agents in those cans that can separate the non-stick surface on your air fryer basket. In this way, if you need to splash foods directly in the basket, invest in a hand-pumped kitchen spray bottle.

- Use the proper breading procedure. Breading is an imperative way in many air fryer recipes. Do not avoid a stage! It is vital to coat food with flour in the first place, at that point egg and after that the breadcrumbs. Be tenacious about the breadcrumbs and press them onto the food with your hands. Because the air fryer has a strong fan as a component of its instrument, breading can sometimes blow off the food. Pressing those morsels on immovably will enable the breading to adhere.

➤ Use an aluminum foil sling. Getting extra pieces into and out of the air fryer basket can be dubious. To make it easier, crease a bit of aluminum foil into a strip about 2-inches wide by 24-inches long. Place the cake container or baking dish on the foil and by holding the closures of the foil, you will be ready to lift the skillet or dish and lower it into the air fryer basket. Overlap or tuck the finishes of the aluminum foil into the air fryer basket, and after that return the basket to the air fryer. When you are prepared to evacuate the dish, unfurl and grab the ends of the aluminum foil to lift the pan out of the air fryer basket.

Click here to check out the rest of (**Air Fryer Cookbook: Easy to Cook Delicious Air Fryer Recipes**) on Amazon.

Check Out My Other Books

Below you'll find some of my other popular books that are popular on Amazon

and Kindle as well. Simply click on the links below to check them out.

Alternatively, you can visit my author page on Amazon to see other work done by

me.

<u>Paleo Diet: Paleo Diet Recipes for Healthy Weight Loss</u>

 If the links do not work, for whatever reason, you can simply search for these

titles on the Amazon website to find them.